OUR JOURNEY THROUGH ALZHEIMER'S

One Caregiver's Story

Dorothy C. Snyder

This book is a work of non-fiction. Names and places have been changed to protect the privacy of all individuals. The events and situations are true.

ISBN: 1-4140-3230-7 (e-book)
ISBN: 1-4140-3229-3 (Paperback)

This book is printed on acid free paper.

1stBooks – rev. 11/21/03

For my four wonderful children,
Susan, Karen, Richard and Brad,
who were with me throughout this journey.

With Love,
Mom

ACKNOWLEDGMENTS

It would be impossible to thank each person individually who accompanied me on this caregiving journey.

In particular though I wish to thank my church family who was there for me through the long months and years. Without them I could not have made it through.

A big thank you to my support group who inspired and encouraged me by listening to me vent and giving me hugs when I needed them most.

I extend special thanks to my editor, Nina Anderson, who encouraged me to write my story and edited my words so they were readable.

And finally, my children who were with me the whole time and shared the pain and sorrow.

Contents

Preface

~~~~~~~

I walked a mile with sorrow,
and ne'er a word said she.
But oh, the things I learned from her
when sorrow walked with me.
- Robert Browning

Caregiving is much like parenting; little, if any, training, is given for either.

On-the-job training is how we learn to cope. Sadly, once we have gained this knowledge, whether it is parenting or caregiving, there is little use for either. Young parents prefer to learn from their own experience, and the caregiver is usually in denial about what is happening. Rosalynn Carter in her book, *"Helping Yourself Help Others"*, says it best, "We learn about the caregiving role only when we actually have to take it on, and then we need a road map."

I hope that by writing about our experience, other caregivers who are beginning the Alzheimer's journey will be encouraged from reading our story.

Even though things may seem overwhelming, I would like you to know you can do it. You are equal to the task and you are not alone. There are others who understand and are willing to help.

Strength and power can be gained as we encounter others who have experienced situations similar to our own. There is strength in numbers, and when we realize that our suffering is not unique to us, it becomes more bearable. A sorrow (or pain) shared is a sorrow divided, and hopefully my account will give other caregivers hope and comfort in the face of their pain.

Family and friends walked with us and when we grew weary, they were there with loving support. Because of such help, I feel it is important that families acknowledge the illness and explain it to others. More importantly though, God accompanied us on each painful step through what has been called the "long goodbye."

Having taken this journey with a loved one, I feel I must make my pain pay dividends or it will have been for nothing. What better way than to "comfort those in any trouble with the same comfort we ourselves have received from God."
(2 Corinthians 1: 3-4)

Making myself available to others who are experiencing this painful disease and being there with a sympathetic ear, hugs when needed, and a comforting word, is but a small way in which I can pay back for the help I so generously received from family and friends. Telling our story is another way I hope to encourage those who are either on the journey now or who will be facing it in the future

Chapter One

Diagnosis

~~~~~

***You don't have to see the whole staircase,
just take the first step.***
—Martin Luther King, Jr.

When Herrick and I decided to take early
retirement we thought we had all the time we needed
for the activities we had put on hold to raise our family
and secure our future. Little did we know that on our
first trip following retirement, there would be signs
that all was not quite right.

I tucked my suspicions and fears in a back corner
of my mind, telling myself he was just tired and that
was the reason for my husband's confusion and
irritability, even though he was one who was always
optimistic and never had a down day.

Following our return home there were incidents of
'lost' items such as tools and keys, and other troubling
behaviors. While I was puzzled about this behavior, I
still was not concerned enough to seek help.

After a few months, I finally asked our primary
care physician about the behaviors I was noticing. His
reply was, "Oh, that is just the way your husband is
aging. We all go through similar things."

I should not have let his comment lull me into wasting a whole year before seeking specialized help. Never, EVER let a doctor put you off if you notice something which you know is not quite right. You know your loved one, and yourself, better than anyone else can.

When we finally consulted a neurologist, every conceivable test was made to determine if something physical might be causing these strange behaviors. This was in the mid-90's and except for President Reagan's letter disclosing he had Alzheimer's, there was little publicity about this debilitating disease. When nothing physical was uncovered, extensive psychological tests were given.

Our visit with the doctor following completion of these tests is as vivid today as it was on that late May afternoon. A kind and gentle man, the doctor told us that in his opinion he was 95% certain my husband suffered from mild to moderate Alzheimer's disease.

Just as we are all different individuals, our reactions to news of this scope will be different. Herrick and I were in shock and asked the doctor no questions, just walked out and went to our car. After getting into the car, my husband said, "This should not be happening to you." His thoughts were totally for me and how this was going to impact my future, giving no immediate thought to his. We held onto each other and cried for a few minutes before driving home

My husband's diagnosis was prior to any medicines being on the market for Alzheimer's and we had no options for slowing the progress of the disease. Thankfully, there are several drugs available today, which will slow the progression of the disease, letting the patient continue a normal lifestyle for a longer period of time.

I am confident that as time goes by, more medicines will become available. The earlier a diagnosis can be made, the sooner medical intervention can begin. Maximizing function and quality of life for the longest period of time should be your goal for your loved one.

From the start, the children and I decided we would share the diagnosis with our extended family, our friends, and our church. We knew even then that we could not do this alone, but would need help and support. Like any other decision in life, this is a personal one, and there is no absolute right or wrong decision. However, I do not advise anyone to try to walk a solitary path through the pain of Alzheimer's disease.

If I had known on that beautiful May afternoon what lay ahead for us on our journey through Alzheimer's disease, I might have become discouraged or depressed, but I do not believe I would have done a single thing differently.

Taking one day at a time is all one can do anyway, so fretting and buying into the future prevents us from living today to its fullest. The thing to remember is that we do what we know how to do, to the best of our ability, then leave the rest to God.

Beginning the very day of the doctor's frightening diagnosis, I began keeping a journal, one of the wisest things I did for myself. On those blank pages I could pour out my pain, anger and frustration, and even ask questions. And, yes, there were times I did question God. My journal was my confidant and my friend.

As I watched my husband struggling to make sense of this strange and frightening world to which the disease had taken him, it took all my will power to stay centered and focused on the day to day duties. The journal helped me to do this.

Keeping a daily journal is one of the first things I suggest to new caregivers in the support group which I co-facilitate. A few minutes writing in your journal each day will go a long way in helping you cope.

Writing down your feelings helps sort through the tangle of emotions. As you put words to your feelings, you can understand yourself better

Chapter 2

ACCEPTANCE

~~~~~~

Denial is the innocents way of putting off until tomorrow what hurts too much to accept today.
—Unknown

I went through the stages of despair, anger and denial before finally coming to accept that my husband's problem was not curable, nor at that time, even treatable. The grief experienced is not unlike that of grief over the death of someone you love.

Though all indications pointed to nothing except Alzheimer's disease being responsible for my husband's mental problems, I still clung to the hope that another, treatable explanation would be found. His doctors were kind and understanding as I called again and again imploring them to run "just one more test."

And while my dear husband was long suffering and would go along with each rabbit I thought we should chase, I realize you may be dealing with someone who will not even go for the initial tests, much less consent to continued testing.

The only suggestion I can offer, if you are experiencing this problem, is that you keep trying. If possible, get family members, clergy and your family doctor to intervene and try to convince your loved one to go for testing and diagnosis. The sooner you know for sure, the earlier you can begin treatment, if indicated.

Once the diagnosis was made, I began gathering information on the disease from every source I could find. The local Alzheimer's Association was the first place I started. They will provide educational information, as well as information on the local support groups in your area. I found their personnel to be knowledgeable, caring and supportive. If you cannot find one in your local area, there is a national organization who will assist you.

If you have access to the internet, there are many sites where you can go for information, most of which is free of charge.

There is an old German adage which says, "Knowledge is power." Nowhere does this have more meaning than for those caring for a loved one with Alzheimer's disease.

Being informed is being prepared to face reality. Knowing what to expect can take some of the fear and uncertainty out of the journey. Joining a local support group is a great source of strength. Having someone to share experiences with can relieve some of the stress. There are even online support groups for those who have internet available to them.

Beginning with your local library all the way to the

internet, you can find books on Alzheimer's disease, as well as caregiving in general. One book I found especially helpful was *The 36-Hour Day* by Nancy L. Mace and Peter V. Rabins. But it is not a book I could take in all at once. Only as changes took place with my husband was I able to go to the book to see what was written about any new behavior.

Checking references only as a new situation arose was my way of keeping a distance between that which I knew in my heart would be coming and still be able to cope with what was happening in the present.

The point is, be as informed as you can and you will feel more in control.

From despair to denial, then finally acceptance can be a long journey. Coming to accept the diagnosis was a fearful, isolating time for Herrick and me. Family and friends were there to embrace us and offer encouragement, but when we were alone it was as though we were in a fearful country with no compass to guide us. The loss of the companionship of my husband only intensified my loneliness.

The first few years were worse for Herrick than for me as he still understood some of what was happening to him. The latter stages of the disease were worse for me as I watched helplessly the almost daily losses he experienced.

Early in the journey after accepting the diagnosis, I learned the wisdom of taking one day at a time.

Trying to look to the future and think about what we would be facing months or years down the road was too depressing. I learned to leave the future in God's hands.

Chapter 3

Finding Joy in the Journey

~~~~~~~~~

"Life isn't a matter of milestones, but of moments"
-Rose Fitzgerald Kennedy

Once we had accepted the inevitable, we made the decision to take life one day at a time and to make each day count. Storing up memories was a gift we could give ourselves .We knew we could not lose any of the precious time we had left.

Finding something Herrick could enjoy each day became my daily goal. We had always enjoyed eating out, especially trying any new restaurant opening in our area. So we continued doing this, making it a weekly event. As the disease worsened, he was unable to understand the menu and would ask me to order for him or he might tell the waitress to give him what I was having.

Taking walks and identifying wildflowers and birds was something we had always enjoyed, so as weather permitted we continued to take our walks. Forgetting the names of familiar items was worse for him on some days, but we never let that stop us from continuing our routine.

Attending Sunday School and church was a lifetime habit and we continued going. The time came

9

when regularly attending both services became too much for him. We stopped going to Sunday School and attended worship service only. He loved to sing and when it became impossible for him to follow the words in hymnals, he would sing from memory or hum along.

Listening to television or music on CD's or the radio was also something he enjoyed. Once as he was listening to a favorite performer singing, he remarked, "This is the best ever!" He was still able to find pleasure in the things he had always enjoyed.

By the next morning he would have forgotten our trip to the movies or to a concert, but the pleasure he received while at the movie or concert made the trip worthwhile.

You know your loved ones better than anyone else. Involve them in activities which you know brought joy in the past. Keep to your normal routine as much as your loved ones can or wants to. You will know from their reactions if it is not pleasing them. Do not wait for their input or suggestions for things to do, as they are either unsure of their judgment or too confused to remember what they like to do.

The walks may not be as far or as fast, and the words and tunes to the songs may not be exactly right, but who cares? Keep walking and keep singing as long as you can.

With all the dark spots in this long, sad, slow

process, you can find bright spots. And, like the last brilliant rays of the setting sun, the last days are some of the best in my picture book of beautiful memories from my 55 years with Herrick. Just as the last colorful display before the sun sets is more beautiful than the full sunlight of the day, those memories are the ones I treasure and remember the most.

One such moment was the Sunday when our daughter came to stay with her father, while I went to church. I was dressed for church and in the process of getting things arranged for her, when he said to me, "You are the most beautiful thing I have ever seen." Telling me I was lovely and that I looked nice was something he had done throughout our marriage, but this was so totally sincere, so different from husbandly flattery, I was overwhelmed. This comment was one of the best gifts he could have given me

On this journey we must find humor or we will have a tough time enduring. Some of the altered perceptions caused by the disease will give rise to many shared laughs, so relish each one.

One such instance for us was the day when I had laid out Herrick's clothes for him and he walked into the kitchen where I was preparing breakfast wearing his under shorts on top of his pants. I did a double take, then began laughing. He wasn't really sure what amused me, but he began laughing with me.

Not wanting to cause him embarrassment, I refrained from saying a thing about his unusual dress until after we had finished breakfast. Then I suggested we find another color pants for him to wear with the shirt before we went out to our local store. He went along with the suggestion without ever knowing what he had done.

Such events as this can be laughed off easily, while some of the things said or done in public can be more challenging. But it is important that nothing be said or done to cause your loved one to feel unacceptable or ashamed.

I read somewhere that happiness is not a constant state, but isolated moments here and there. We managed to find those moments and they are precious memories.

Sitting on the deck in the late afternoon holding hands and watching the dog play in the yard, or watching the boats on the lake are but two of the many moments we shared, and which are now precious memories. And old memories, like old friends, should be cherished and kept close to our hearts because they are irreplaceable.

Look for and create as many memories as you can in the early part of the Alzheimer's journey. Spend as much time together as you can and you will be amazed at how much closer you become as you accept the inevitable and choose to make the most of it.

It was always a good day and worth every tiring moment when he told me he loved me. Even in his worst moods, he was able to dig deep and find empathy and love for me when he recognized my needs. Brief flashes of the "real" person could surface at any moment. Walking into the room where he lay one day he greeted me with, "Good morning, Good Looking."

Alzheimer's disease may steal your loved one's memories, but it cannot steal the memories you store up during the journey. Start early to collect as many as you can. View these as pearls strung on an unbreakable chain of love.

Chapter 4

The Changing Behavior

~~~~~~

Determine that the thing can and
shall be done, and then we shall find the way.
-Abraham Lincoln

One day when Herrick was depressed and sat and
cried, I asked what was wrong. He told me he did not
know who he was and asked, "What is wrong with
me?" I sat down beside him, held his hand and told
him his name and the names of our four children.
Then I told him I loved him and that he was important
to me and the family. I also told him that God loved
him and cared about all of us. His response was, "Oh,
good. I don't have to cry anymore."

After he had settled down I found a quiet place and
sobbed for him and what he had lost.

I did not try to explain to him what was wrong.
Once before when he had asked what was wrong, and I
had explained about the disease, he told me to just give
him his gun so he could shoot himself.

In the beginning he had listened to what the doctors
told him and understood the diagnosis, but he would
never discuss it with me. If a television program came
on talking about Alzheimer's disease which I wanted
to watch, he would leave the room. Was it too painful
for him to watch? Was he in denial? I do not have the

answer to those questions.

Helping someone come to terms with this disease is good, but only if that person wants to talk about it. If they show no interest, or avoid the subject altogether, what is the purpose? All of us have different ways of coping.

Caregiving is a personal journey. No two are alike, but there are similarities and those are what I would like to touch on in telling our story hoping that in some way it might be of help to others.

In the mid-stage of the disease Herrick's behavior pattern became more off-beat and puzzling. For instance, days on end he would say he needed money or he would ask, "Do we have enough money?" I would assure him that we did have adequate money for our needs, and then I would tell him he had done a great job providing for us. He would thank me, but in a few minutes he would start all over again, saying, "I don't have any money."

One day it dawned on me that perhaps he was wanting some pocket money. I gave him a few dollar bills and a bit of change which he happily put in his pocket and was satisfied.

Trying to figure out where your loved one is in all the tangled perceptions can be frustrating, but keep trying. Once you finally figure out what he/she is trying to express, there is a victory and a joy for you. But more importantly, you have validated your loved one's existence when you show you understand them.

Reasoning with an Alzheimer's patient is impossible. You will be thrown off track again and again by their seeming to be their old selves, then without warning, a response will be uncharacteristically off the wall.

Like the morning Herrick wanted watermelon for breakfast and then refused to eat anything else. Be patient and kind. Act as if this strange request is perfectly logical. Trying to explain that watermelon for breakfast is not reasonable only confuses them more.

As he lost his personality and experienced diminished self-worth, Herrick would say, "I'm no good," or "Just throw me away, I'm not myself anymore." It seemed to me that he was losing his sense of who he was as he realized he could not interact with others as he had always done. At some point Alzheimer's patients understand what is happening and know they are helpless to correct it. Viewed in this light, their anger, hostility and depression is understandable.

Alzheimer's plays havoc with a person's personality. One day my husband would be the sweet, caring, happy man I had married, and the next day he would be a frightened, hostile, angry stranger I did not know.

Learning to separate this stranger from the husband I knew and loved did not happen overnight. A care partner in my support group put it in perspective for me when she suggested I tell myself it was the disease talking and acting this way, not my dear husband. Once I looked at his offensive behavior and language in this light the situation became less stressful for me.

Herrick spoke a great deal about things being lost, or stolen from him. I believe his paranoia about things being stolen came from an awareness that his mind was being taken away, so the only way he could make sense of such a loss was to express fear for his physical possessions.

Losing one's thoughts is difficult, maybe impossible, to articulate, but losing a lawnmower, or having one's car stolen is a concrete loss which can be discussed. That, I think, is the reason for most of the fears my husband had about his possessions being stolen.

Herrick often complained of headaches, saying his eyes hurt. The doctors could find no physical cause. I became aware that these episodes happened most often when he was subjected to emotional stress or mental over-stimulation, which would occur after visits from family or friends. Having him lie down and placing a cool damp cloth over his forehead helped.

As an advocate for your loved one, it is imperative that you control the timing and the length of visits. If you see a visit is upsetting your loved one, say so. Family members and friends will soon get the idea and will know when it is time to leave.

Eventually, your Alzheimer's patient will have to stop driving a car, and this can be a difficult decision. We are, in a way, taking away their independence, and the Alzheimer's patient is going to object. Getting their doctor to inform your loved one that he/she will have to stop driving is one solution. Keeping the car keys hidden is another.

The driving decision was a relatively easy one for us. Our car broke down making it necessary for me buy a new one. Herrick was unable to master the controls on the new car and finally said, "You drive" each time we left the house.

I am not suggesting, of course, that you buy a new car to solve the problem, but anything which works is a solution.

We went through a period when every light in our house had to be turned on. If I turned one off, he would immediately go switch it back on. Was he trying to illuminate his thinking, or was he perhaps afraid and the lights, even during daylight hours, gave him a feeling of security? Like other instances of irrational behavior, I can only speculate.

Many nights he would lie awake in bed and talk to people who had been dead for years, or he would talk about events he thought were going to occur. If I tried to read or sleep he would ask, "Are you listening to me?" His mind would just go on and on because he could not get to sleep, and he did not want me to sleep either.

When I would get so weary I didn't know if I could stand it any longer, I would ask him to please hush and go to sleep. Often he would simply mock me and go right on talking. Going to another room to sleep was not a solution, because he would follow me. When such behavior became so severe I could not function the next day, I hired someone to come in and relieve me so I could rest.

Sleep disturbance builds on itself, creating more problems. Nights with little or no sleep meant confusion, depression and disorientation for Herrick the next day. But if he slept during the day, it meant restlessness that night, and so it went round and round.

The sleep disturbance pattern was hard for me, since most of the time I did not have the luxury of napping during the day. I learned, however, to take every opportunity to rest when he was asleep, even if I didn't go to sleep.

My meticulous husband went for a week one time refusing to take a shower. I found it did not work to try to talk him into taking one, and finally asked my son to try. When he told his father it was time to shower, Herrick willingly went along. By accident, I discovered he was unable to control the water temperature and that seemed to be part of the problem. After I began helping him by adjusting the water temperature, it helped some.

When I asked the doctor about Herrick's reluctance to bathe, his comment was, "I have never known anyone to die from not getting a daily shower or bath; just don't worry so much about it."

After this incident and others similar to it, I learned to relax and let go of things which were not life threatening.

Forgetting how to dress and decisions as simple as which shoe goes on which foot, or leaving the shower and going into the bedroom without drying off and just standing lost in the middle of the room, are just a few of the bizarre behaviors which became routine for us. The sequence of familiar actions is lost and the Alzheimer's patients are unsure of what to do next.

Experiencing the changes we see taking place in the person we love, and watching the person we once knew, become the person we now see, can be frustrating and anxiety producing to say the least. Dealing with these changes takes an immense amount of love and patience on the part of the caregiver.

Coming to terms with the fact that you are now dealing with an adult whose behavior has become much like a child, is not easy. Making the adjustment from the person we once knew to the person our loved one is becoming is difficult. Keeping in mind that the changes must be so much worse for our loved ones as they regress into the sea of dementia will help us keep it in perspective.

As the changes in personality, behavior and physical abilities began to accelerate, my husband began to need and want to go to bed earlier and earlier. There were days when he would be in bed by 6:00 P.M. and want me to go with him. I would get him ready and settled in, then try to do the household chores, or watch the news, but invariably he would get out of bed and hunt for me asking when I was coming to bed. His requests would continue until I gave in and went to bed and read. He was satisfied and comforted by my nearness.

I believe he was either lonely or afraid, perhaps both. Going to bed early was no big sacrifice for me, but just one more adjustment I had to make. Also, it was one more indication that I had no life of my own, apart from that of a caregiver.

Finally the situation developed to the point that he did not want me even reading while he was awake. He seemed to need my undivided attention, as if my very presence was all that gave him a hold on reality. More often than not I would fall asleep as soon as he did because neither of us got more than a couple hours sleep at a stretch. Even when I was asleep, I would be alert to his every move so I could be aware if he left the bed.

These kinds of things were minor compared to his wanting to go "home." Not recognizing our house as his home anymore, he constantly asked to "go home." If I didn't take him in the car and drive around for a while, he would get out of the house and start walking up our driveway by himself.

One day I left him sitting in the den watching TV with his dog Skippy on his lap. I was gone for less than five minutes working in the back part of the house. When I returned to the room, his chair was empty and Skippy was sitting at the back door. I knew Herrick had left the house and immediately began looking around outside, calling to him, but received no response. Walking up to the road, I saw him heading back toward our house.

When I asked him where he had been going he said, "I don't know. I guess I am losing my mind." He knew something terrible was happening to him, but couldn't understand what it was.

Wandering and trying to "go home" is not unusual behavior for those with Alzheimer's disease. There are different opinions as to why they do this, but I think my husband was trying to get back to the life he remembered before the confusion caused by the disease.

There were times he would try to leave the house to find "Mom" or his sister Irene, mumbling, "I'm leaving, they are trying to hurt me." I was never able to figure out who it was he thought was trying to hurt him. I did not try to reason with him by saying there was no one trying to hurt him, but instead assured him I would not let anyone hurt him anymore. He would thank me and be content to come back inside the house.

Slowly, he lost the ability to remember how to do the smallest household chores such as emptying the trash, drying the dishes or even remembering where things were stored. He made no comment at all when I sold the lawn mower and made arrangements to have the lawn work done. Working in the yard had been one of the things he had always enjoyed doing.

In the early days of the disease, when he forgot how to start the lawn mower or the leaf blower, I helped him get it started, then he could do the work on his own. I always stayed outside with him, never leaving him alone while the mower was running.

Letting him continue these activities as long as possible let him feel useful and I am convinced kept the disease at bay a bit longer than if we had given up and not tried to stay active. Staying mentally alert as long as possible by continuing familiar tasks is a must.

He was always able to pick up on my moods. If I became anxious or worried, he sensed it and would be restless and fretful. If I was upbeat and happy, he would be, too. So I began to watch myself, and even on my "bad days" I tried to put on a front to keep him from becoming anxious.

If we are tuned in to their moods, it makes sense that they can pick up on ours. And while it isn't possible to always be happy, making an effort to do so can make a difference in their behavior.

Chapter 5

Caring for the Caregiver

~~~~~~~~

"We all have reservoirs of strength to draw
upon, of which we do not dream"
-William James

Looking back on my life I can see that God prepared me for helping Herrick. All my life I had been caring for someone. First I helped my Mom care for younger siblings. Then a younger sister came to live with me after I was married. My husband's nephew lived with us and attended elementary school for four years. Finally, I cared for an elderly grandmother-in-law for ten years

The only ability God requires is availability, and it seemed I was always the one available. You may be feeling that way, too. Be careful though, because it is all too easy to drift into a "poor me" frame of mind, and such thinking does no one any good. I learned that first hand.

There were nights after my husband had gone to sleep when I would cry and ask God, "Why us, Lord?" Sometimes I wondered if there was no end to my tears. At times I felt my life was out of control, as though I was on a merry-go-round and not able to get off.

Emotional turmoil seems to be our constant companion as we watch our loved ones decline day by day, and it is all too easy to sink into self-pity.

When I began feeling overwhelmed, I knew it was time to hire help so I could take some time off. You will know when it is time to ask for help. And please remember it is not a sign of weakness to do so.

Those who care for a loved one with Alzheimer's disease face a long series of losses as the disease unfolds. As caregivers we must recognize our own grief reactions and find ways to deal with the emotional challenges we will face as these losses occur.

The mood swings the disease causes our loved ones to experience leaves us the caregiver struggling to stay on an even keel. And feeling sorry for them does not make it any easier for us. Is it any wonder that we find ourselves crying and feeling moody?

One moment my husband might say, "Get the h--- away from me!", and in almost the same breath say something like "You're pretty and I love you."

Did I hug him enough and tell him often enough that I loved him? Such questions will come and it is only human that they do. The important thing to remember is we do the best we know how with our limited knowledge of the situation.

Harboring a "poor me" mind set got me nowhere. Only as I found purpose was I able to shrug off that self destructive feeling. I learned to focus on Herrick and his needs. Did I sacrifice some part of my life in order to do this? Of course, I did.

But with every sacrifice I found a corresponding compensation. For instance, the need to be at home with him made it necessary that I drop out of outside activities. With this extra time, my love of flowers led me into pressing flowers, designing and creating note cards, an activity I still enjoy.

My love of reading helped me to connect with my husband by reading to him, but also led me to writing for publication. These were activities I could enjoy and still be at home with him.

If we are to have anything of substance to offer to those we are caring for, we must first take time for our own renewal.

A dear friend who is now experiencing this same restriction on outside activities is becoming more and more involved with quilting. Quilting was something she had dabbled in previously, but now finds great satisfaction in creating lovely quilts for her own use, and as gifts, while being at home with her husband.

I urge you to find a hobby or craft which you can enjoy and do at home. This hobby, or activity, will be the outlet you go to time and time again for a feeling of fulfillment and satisfaction. A brief time of reading or meditating may be just what you need for a short respite. Dr. Wayne Dyer in his book. *Your Sacred Self,* says, "To avoid being consumed by anything, you must be able to walk away from it."

The advice usually given caregivers about caring for themselves is how important it is to keep physically fit. And certainly exercise, good nutrition and adequate rest are vitally important. Becoming physically exhausted would do no one any good. However, there is more involved than just staying physically fit.

We are more than one dimensional beings. We are body, mind and spirit. What good is keeping ourselves together physically if we fall apart emotionally and spiritually?

Caregiving engages a person's whole being, and a significant part of our being is spiritual. When we do not refuel spiritually, it does not take long for us to become spiritually bankrupt. Shortly thereafter comes lack of peace and feelings of being depressed and unable to cope.

We each must find our own way for refueling spiritually. For me, it was finding regular times for Bible reading, prayer and meditation. Also, I found great comfort and peace in short walks or sitting for a while on the outside deck just absorbing the beauty of nature. Listening to quiet music was not only refreshing for me but my husband enjoyed it also.

Never give up on your quiet time. Quiet, relaxing moments keep us focused and able to find meaning in what we are doing. There are no saints among us. We need to realize we are human and doing the very best we can.

Caregiving is a hard job both physically and mentally and we need to acknowledge our limits and know when to ask for help.

If you find yourself becoming irritated over small things, your eating habits are changing drastically, or you have trouble sleeping, please reach out for help. Perhaps you should consult your physician.

If family or friends cannot give you the respite you need, consider hiring someone to come in nights so you can get a full night's rest. Caregiver burnout is common and it will not help your loved one if you let this happen. Getting inadequate rest is always a danger.

Emotions are natural, human responses; they are neither right nor wrong, good or bad. Be honest about your feelings. Express how you feel. Sometimes a good hard cry can bring relief and peace to your soul.

No matter how overwhelming all this sounds, you can navigate the journey. Just take it one day at a time.

Chapter 6

Through Difficult Times

~~~~~

Things work out best for those
who make the best of the way things are.
-Anonymous

Just when I thought my life could not get any more complicated, something would happen which proved me wrong. At this stage of our journey there were painful incidents, which represent some of the common experiences you may face. It is my hope that by sharing them, you will be able to discover ways of coping with and better understand difficult behavior.

Everyone is unique, but there are similarities with which you can connect. At the very least, please remember always that you are not alone on this journey.

Problems with incontinence began in the mid-stage of the disease. In the beginning, he would always apologize for causing me the trouble of having to care for him. My heart broke to have this stalwart man on whom I had leaned for so many years saying, "I'm sorry" and have tears in his eyes as he endured my caring for him in this intimate manner. Showing understanding and being patient in these situations made it easier for him to maintain his dignity. We treated it in as "matter of fact" manner as possible.

The extra work and the constant grief of caring for a loved one with dementia requires resilience. Simply coming to terms with the losses my husband was suffering was so stressful that at times I didn't think I could bear it. But bear it, I did and so can you.

I found it is true that we do find strength we never dreamed we had when faced with situations where our loved one needs our strength. We find not only physical strength, but emotional and spiritual as well.

Betty Ford has been quoted as saying, "We never know how much strength we have until we have to use it."

Three years following the diagnosis of Alzheimer's, Herrick suffered a major stroke which caused physical disability. Whether the stroke was a result of the disease, the doctors could not say. After several months of therapy he was finally able to walk again with the aid of a walker and/or walking cane.

Physical therapy was agony for him as he did not always understand directions from the therapist. He would become frustrated and say unkind things to her. She shrugged them off and kept urging him to take another step or push a little harder—whatever it was she was asking him to do. She did not give up until he was able to walk on his own with the aid of a cane or walker.

During therapy, it became obvious that further mental deterioration had occurred. Impossible to say whether it was a result of the stroke or simply the progression of the disease, but his ability to understand what was being said had declined.

Reading the newspaper or watching television no longer interested him. In both instances, they provided too much information for him to take in. Also, any program he saw on television involving violence or crime upset him terribly. He took it all personally.

There were nights, after he had gone to sleep, when I would lie beside him crying, and ask God "Why?" Some days I wondered if I would be able to hold on for the long haul. Like David in Psalm 22:1, there were times I felt like crying out, "My God, my God, why have you forsaken me?"

Yet even when I felt deserted, God's promise that he would never leave me if I trusted in Him, enabled me to hang on and keep going. Even though resolved not to let things upset me, I am human. There were times when I would be tired and just could not help becoming upset.

Once when I had gone grocery shopping and left Herrick with a sitter, he needed to go to the bathroom but would not tell the sitter, so he had an accident. While undressing and showering him and cleaning the bathroom floor, I began to cry. He looked at me and asked, "Don't you like me anymore?" Then he said, "Don't cry, give me a kiss."

I was always amazed, that even in his disease

confused mind, his love for me was strong enough to surface when he saw me distressed. Always he would try to comfort me. Such times hurt on many levels.

Our loved ones do still care about us, they just can't understand, and do not know how to express their feelings.

With each loss my husband suffered, I suffered for him. The day he walked into the kitchen where I was preparing lunch, and asked, "Who am I?" was one of the worst times. After answering him as calmly as I could manage and hearing his quiet, "Thank you" I went into the bathroom and sobbed. It was evident that the disease had finally robbed him of who he was.

Some days he would be pleasant with the sitter who came twice weekly for a few hours. Other days he would be irritable and angry with her and with me for leaving him. When he was upset and irritable he would not eat. Like dealing with a child, I would have to coax him to eat and finally he would. I was afraid at these times that he was experiencing pain but was not able to tell me.

When I would comment on having to walk the dog, or load the washer, he would volunteer to help me. One time, as I have recorded in my journal, he said, "I love you, won't you let me help you?" Again, his true self would emerge from the confusion and shine through at the most unexpected moments

Since it is impossible to know just how much an

Alzheimer's patient is capable of understanding, I wonder if I was right to put him off and not be totally honest when he would ask me questions.

Two questions he asked more than once were, "What is wrong with me?" and "Why can't I get better?" Instead of telling him he would never get better, I told him he had a disease and the doctors were treating him.

Was I wrong in not being totally truthful? Would I have been doing him a favor by telling him he would only get worse? I don't think so, but each of us must decide which answers work. My rational mind knows he would not have understood, nor would he have found comfort in my answer if I had gone into detail.

What purpose can possibly be gained by causing more pain and stress by talking about the inevitable? Sometimes we can show love by telling a white lie and sparing unnecessary pain. However, you know your loved one better than anyone else, so go with your gut instinct if questioned.

Once when he asked , "Why me?" I told him I did not know but God knew. He said, "We'll be all right then." And almost immediately he said "Remember, I don't want you to cry, I'll be with you." I believe he knew and understood that he would most likely die before I did.

Chapter 7

Making the Best of It

~~~~~~

***Things work out best for those who make the
best of the way things are.***
-Anonymous

The inconsistent behavior of a person with
Alzheimer's disease is one of the hardest situations for
the caregiver. The emotional impact is enormous.
Because we are human it is not always possible to
remember that it is the disease and not our loved one,
who is speaking or acting unkindly. Often we will
react in the same manner.

One time in particular I remember yelling at
Herrick because of something he had done.
Immediately, I began crying because I knew I should
not have yelled at him. He apologized and said, "I do
the best I can. Please stop crying."

Remembering such incidents is painful. But it will
happen every now and then. Just don't beat yourself
up when it does.

Jekell and Hyde personalities emerge from the
Alzheimer's damaged brain at the most unexpected
times. We would be going along on a fairly even keel,
then out of the blue Herrick would do or say something
totally out of character. One moment he would tell me

how much he appreciated everything I did for him, then turn right around and tell me to leave him alone, that he could do very well without me.

One time he told me to just throw him out; he was no good to anyone anymore. What a confusing world it must have been for him to know he was not in control of his actions, but still able to understand some of the things he did was wrong. As caregivers, we hurt when we see such agonizing and frightening confusion overtake our loved ones.

I know that on some level Herrick remembered and understood when he had been in one of his hostile, ugly moods. It was not at all unusual for him to say, "I was just dizzy," which I understood was his way of apologizing and trying to communicate to me how mixed up he felt.

Showing love and compassion gets awfully hard when an Alzheimer's patient's behavior is anything but loving. Counting to ten and remembering it is the disease causing the behavior will pull you through.

It was painful, but also reassuring, when Herrick talked about his love for me and the family. He would say, "How good it is," wanting, I believe, to be reassured we would always be together. Then in the blink of an eye, he would become hostile, asking where were we, and when were we going home. I came to realize he was afraid when these moods struck.

Everything, even our home, eventually became unfamiliar to him.

Many times I could reassure him and get him settled down, but as often as not, it would take an antidepressant, which the doctor had prescribed for just such times. It pays to keep in close touch with your primary care physician or neurologist, who will be able to help you in such situations.

Herrick never refused to take medicines from me, but he refused to take them from anyone else. He never lost his trust in me for which I am enormously grateful.

There are instances when getting medications taken in a timely manner can be challenging. Ask the doctor or nurse for suggestions when your loved one resists taking medications. I found it worked best for us if I crushed a pill and put it in applesauce or some other food, but this works only when pills can be crushed. Always check with your doctor or pharmacist before crushing any pills. Some medications might be the time-release kind and crushing would not be good.

Following Herrick's stroke the episodes of hallucinations really accelerated. Coming into a room and finding him having a conversation with someone visible only to him was not unusual. I learned it did no good to tell him there was no one sitting in the chair in the corner. His perceptions were real to him. Eventually I learned to take it in stride and go where he was in his reality. To have me participate was

39

reassuring to him.

A sense of humor can brighten almost anything you encounter. Billy Graham had it right when he said, "A keen sense of humor helps us to overlook the unbecoming, understand the unconventional, overcome the unexpected and outlast the unbearable."

Many times being able to laugh saved awkward situations from being embarrassing or hurtful for us. When we understand the reasons for strange behaviors, it is easier to handle them. Lighten up, find a sense of humor and you will find more joy in the journey.

My daily goal was to make Herrick's day as peaceful and joyful for him as I possibly could. Posted on my refrigerator door was the saying ancient Greeks used to whisper to each other every morning: "When shall we live if not today." That became my motto, as I learned to live in the present and not look to the future.

In spite of the circumstances, we can find happiness if we let ourselves. An anonymous saying, "Life is not measured by the number of breathes we take, but by the moments that take our breath away" is so true.

Chapter 8

The Mountain Gets Steeper

~~~~~~

I prayed that God would remove this mountain
from my path; instead He gave me the strength to climb
it..
-Unknown

Easter Sunday two years before his death was the last time my husband was able to attend church services. His comment as we were leaving was, "I like this church. Can we come again?" This was the church where he was a member for 28 years. The church in which he had served as Deacon, and eventually the church in which his memorial service would be held.

Even though all previous memories of attending church in that place had been erased by Alzheimer's disease, he still found acceptance and peace.

We never know how much an Alzheimer's patient can remember, but we do know feelings and emotions are still sensitive, which is why they react to our moods, and can feel our love. And, why it is so important that we continue to let them know they are loved and remain an important part of our lives.

In addition to the sitter who came twice weekly, I eventually hired a housekeeper who came two hours twice a week to help with the housework and stay with my husband so I could get a break. He didn't mind her being around if I was also present, but resented my absence when I left the house, becoming moody and uncooperative.

His moodiness was so childlike that just as we used to do with our children when they were small, I would leave the house without his knowing I was going. The passage of time had no meaning for him. I could be away for two hours or for only twenty minutes and it was all the same for him. Each time I entered the room, he would greet me as if I had been gone for hours, asking, "Where have you been? I've missed you."

This type of behavior reflected the loneliness, fright and the loss he was feeling. Since I was the constant in his life he probably felt I was abandoning him. Not being able to understand the passage of time he may have thought I was going for good. I finally realized he was not being manipulative—as I first thought—but was expressing his feelings the only way he knew how.

It is astonishing that Alzheimer's disease can reduce our strong, self-reliant loved ones to the state of behaving like a child. But it can.

Once when he spit his pills out, and I asked him why he had done it, his response was, "Because you told me to." Apparently, when I had asked him to swallow, he had understood me to say "spit." The doctor had warned me that his perception of the spoken word might get so mixed up he would have problems understanding. Perceiving things in reverse was not unusual for him.

I learned it is important to speak slowly and use as few words as possible. I found it helpful if Herrick looked directly at me when I spoke to him.

To get my attention, he would yell, "Help me" each time I got out of his sight. When I asked what was wrong, he would say he wanted me to stay in the room with him. He apparently was afraid to be alone, and needed me in his sight to help him hold on to whatever reality he had. The need to have me in his sight continued only for a few weeks, then we moved on to something else.

I cannot emphasis enough that it is important to go where they are in their delusions. When Herrick saw a man sitting in the corner of our bedroom one night, instead of trying to tell him there was no one there, I asked if we knew him. Or when he told me he had just come home from visiting his mother (who had been dead for over 25 years), I asked if it had been a good visit.

When Alzheimer's patients are having these delusions, that is their reality, and we only confuse them further by trying to reason with them. Instead, validate their reality.

Those suffering from Alzheimer's can easily become overwhelmed. The logical, reasoning, and problem solving parts of the brain are the first to be affected by the disease. Only the primitive parts of the brain are left to control behavior, which leads to fear and aggression. No wonder our loved ones lash out in frustration and anger.

Whether a result of the stroke or simply deterioration from the disease, I do not know, but Herrick began going into coma-like sleep patterns. He would be impossible to wake up. His breathing would be shallow, and at times he would wave his hands around, but would not respond to my calling his name, shaking him, or even washing his face with a cold towel.

The first two or three times this happened—once mid-morning, the other times at night—I called 911 and had him transported to the emergency room. Testing for further strokes showed nothing, and after a few hours he would again be alert. The only reason given by the doctors for these deep coma-like sleep patterns, was "possible TIA's." I was told there was no reason to bring him to the hospital when they occurred. One doctor told me not to be surprised if it began to happen more frequently..

Before I could get comfortable with one change, it seemed another would occur. As a caregiver friend said to me, "Caregiving is like a game of golf: you get out of one hole just to get in another." Learning to be resilient is a must, and being resilient is easier if you can get adequate rest.

Once I realized I was trying to control Herrick's

schedule of waking, sleeping, eating, and was forcing him to keep to a routine, I began to let him sleep instead of waking him on my schedule. If he was not hungry at regular mealtime, I would let it slide and try again a bit later, which worked for a while.

During the period when sleeping the usual nighttime hours was not happening, he would sleep off and on during the day. I would try to nap or at least rest when he did. As his coma-like nighttime sleep became more frequent, I would often be afraid to sleep for fear I would wake up one morning and find him dead.

The sundowning, or the Sundown Effect referred to by doctors, usually occurred for us in late afternoon. The confusion seems to be a result of overload from the activities and sensory happenings during the day. For Herrick, the sundown confusion usually occurred around 3:00 PM. He would get up and say "I'm going home." I learned to agree with him and we would go for a ride. Most of the time a ride would settle him down. Many times he would recognize our home as we drove back down the driveway, and say "Thank you for bringing me home."

There were times, however, when he refused to get in the car and would start walking. I would walk along with him. Because of the stroke damage, he was unable to walk far without tiring, and I would ask him if he wanted to go back home and let me call someone to come pick us up. He would stop and consider it for a moment and then agree. Most of the time when we got back in the house, he would be perfectly content to let me give him a drink of water, and one of his anti-anxiety pills "while we waited." Usually he fell asleep and would have forgotten all about our walk by the time he woke up.

Trying different activities to take the diseased mind off the desire to wander, whether it is voiced "going home" or just pacing, seems to help. Some-times quiet music, or quiet reading would calm my husband until he fell asleep.

I remember well one dramatic afternoon. Herrick insisted he was going home whether I went with him or not. We started out driving around as usual when he suddenly told me to stop the car, that he was "getting out of here and going home." Instead of calming down as he usually did when I told him we were going home, he became more and more upset and told me that if I didn't take him home he would kill me, then kill himself. He began trying to wrestle the steering wheel from me. When I resisted his efforts he tried to open the door and get out of the moving car, saying "Let me out right now." Luckily, I had put the childproof lock on before we left the house, otherwise I don't think I could have controlled the situation.

That scene was a scary time when I was not sure that I could maintain control. Such episodes were, I believe, his trying to get away from the fears of what was happening to him and to get back to the way he was.

That was the last day I took him for a drive, because I feared for our safety if something like that should happen again.

Chapter 9

Facing our Fears

~~~~~~

*"You gain strength, courage, and confidence
by every experience in which you really stop
to look fear in the face"*
-Eleanor Roosevelt

One entry in my journal almost two years before
Herrick's death reads: "Life goes on, one precious day
after the other. But one day in the not too distant
future it will be over. Is it all right to cry before it
happens? Some days the tears begin without any
thought or provocation. Does an inner knowing sense
the coming events which the conscious mind refuses to
acknowledge?"

There is such a thing as anticipatory grief. When
we think of grief we usually think of the feeling we
experience when a loved one dies. In dealing with a
loved one with Alzheimer's disease, we really begin
this process when that loved one is diagnosed. This
grief is confusing. On one hand our loved one is still
with us, but on the other hand, we have already begun
to grieve their loss.

Losing a loved one is never easy, but having time
to say goodbye is a precious gift. I took the
opportunity to tell my husband I loved him at least
once a day. I sat and talked to him about how much I
appreciated him for all the years he had taken care of

me and the children, and thanked him for being a wonderful husband.

Sometimes when he rambled on about wanting to "go home," I believe he was actually talking about his heavenly home and not the place where he grew up, or even the life he lived prior to the disease. One night when he had been gazing out the window staring into space, he seemed to be "otherworldly" as if he were between earth and heaven. Later that same night I was awakened by his chanting "going home to Jesus."

There were times he would ask, "I didn't kill anyone did I?" Or when a thunder storm raged with loud thunder, he would yell, "Get down, they are shooting at us again!" Or he would wake me up at night saying "Ka boom" as if he were listening to gunfire. I shared these happenings with the Social worker at our local Alzheimer's Association.

A psychologist called me one day saying the local Alzheimer's Association had given her my telephone number—I had given them permission—and she ask if I would mind sharing some of Herrick's behavior with her. She was studying post-traumatic stress syndrome in Alzheimer's patients. She knew my husband had served in the Navy during WW II and thought he might be reliving some of his war experiences.

In her research she had found that many veterans with dementia seemed to be recalling war experiences, especially those who had not consciously processed traumatic war experiences. I don't know if she was right, but I do know Herrick never talked much about his experiences during the war.

I gave the psychologist permission to write an article about Herrick's experience. When the article was published in our local newspaper, I received positive feedback from readers who said the article answered questions about the behavior of their sick veterans.

Being awakened in the night with Herrick having bed shaking chills became common during the last 18 months. He would say, "I'm dying" or "Please help me." I would pile blankets on him, cradle him in my arms and talk soothingly until he became quiet. Often, following one of these episodes he would ask "You will keep me, won't you?" He cried often during these times. Again, his behavior was childlike and reminded me of how our children were when small and had been ill and hurting.

When our out-of-town children came to visit and stayed in the house, he became fretful and hard to get along with. I thought it was because he was resentful of my attention being taken from him. In retrospect, however, I believe it was because of the extra noise and changes in the routine.

Any time our loved ones cannot understand and follow what is happening around them, it causes overload and the result is irritability. Keeping them in their comfort zone as much as possible is always best. You will quickly understand what upsets your loved one and causes irritability.

As Herrick lost the ability to remember who I was, he would often resent my doing things for him. A totally new personality would emerge and he would tell me to leave, that he could do fine without me. Or, who did I think I was anyway? Sure, on some level it hurt, but when I reminded myself why he was behaving this way, I could cope.

Times when he was somewhat lucid, he would ask, "When am I going to be like others?" or "I want to go home to myself." There were nights when he would be awake for hours, fighting some one, and talking to someone only he could see.

Following such nights it was not unusual for him to say he was going to kill himself. The only gun in the house was his father's old pistol, which I locked away. I had no idea if he really would harm himself, but I was not willing to take a chance.

During this period I recorded in my journal what Calvin Miller had written in **Jesus Loves Me,** "We are all dying on our way to being dead. Dying is not so much a point as it is a process. We do some of it every day until it is all done."

Miller's words brought home to me that while I was grieving what was happening to us personally, our experience was not foreign to the human race as a whole. We are all going through the same thing. It is just a matter of perspective.

The first time Herrick fell was in the middle of the night. He had gotten out of bed and was heading for the bedroom door when I heard him fall and exclaimed, "Oh, no!" He responded instantly telling me he was all right.

That was the beginning of many falls. I began to notice he was gradually becoming weaker. I tried to keep my eye on him each time he got out of his chair or bed. If he fell and my daughter or her husband were not available to help me get him up and back in his chair, I called on neighbors, who were always willing to come at any hour. When he fell, Herrick always assured me that he was all right and for me not to cry. As he had done throughout our 50 plus years of marriage, he would think of me first.

I began to notice that after a sleepless night of "talking to people" he would be more anxious and confused the next day. Some of the people he talked to had names I recognized, but some I had never heard before his nighttime conversations.

One night stands out in my memory. He told me he had been talking with his mother. So I asked if she was still with him. He said no that she had to go be with his brother because he needed her more.

Not more than three weeks following this incident, his brother's 45-year-old daughter was diagnosed with terminal cancer and died not too much longer after that. Whether my husband actually knew of the impending death from communication with his mother, I won't know this side of heaven.

He seemed comfortable with these conversations and would even pause as if listening to someone answering him. Following one such night, the first thing he said the next morning was, "I want to go home to Mommy." I had known him since he was twenty years old and never heard him to call his mother anything but "Mother" or "Mom." The name "Mommy" had to have come from way back in his childhood.

There were times he was loving and wanted to hold me—some of my best memories. His eyes would light up and he would smile when I told him I loved him and that he was important to me and our family. I tried always to remember that the person I was caring for was more important than my caregiving duties. While he may not have understood everything I said or did, he still felt and needed love and encouragement.

The real person, who was my husband of over 50 years and the father of our four children, lived within that confused brain until the day God called him home. I tried never to forgot that, and at least once every day told him I loved him. On good days, he would answer back saying that he loved me, too.

I will be eternally grateful to friends, especially his male friends, who came by and talked to him as if he were not disabled at all. Those visits meant so much to him—and to me. One afternoon following a friend's visit, my husband asked when he was coming again, saying that he wished the friend would come live with us. We should never underestimate how much our staying in touch with others means to them.

Friends did more than visit and pray for us. They showed their love and care in many tangible ways. Loaves of fresh baked bread, vegetables from their garden, and offers to visit with Herrick while I ran errands were just a few of the many ways they showered us with their loving care.

Following a visit from our granddaughter and great granddaughter one day he told me that he loved me and did not want me to cry when he was gone. And then he told me he did not want me to get hurt. His little speech was surprising because by then he was having trouble putting words together to form sentences.

I understood his telling me he did not want me to get hurt was his way of saying that my caring for him at home was not a good idea, and he was afraid I was going to hurt myself. Thoughts like these must have surfaced from deep within and were somehow triggered by having been with the children.

Normal moments such as these are inspiring for caregivers and give us the strength to keep going. They will diminish as the weeks pass, but hang onto them as long as you can. It is comforting to know your loved one experiences good moments even in the midst of their fears and confusion.

Chapter 10

Strength for the Journey

~~~~~~

God Whispers in our pleasures,
but shouts in our pain.
-C. S. Lewis

Inevitably, there comes a time when the painful moments outweigh the pleasurable. Then we realize that if we are to continue in the role of caregiver, we must have strength beyond our own.

I did have faith and continuously reminded myself that I was not alone; God was with me. To keep going I had to believe there was some purpose, or lesson, in what was happening. I still do not understand the purpose for my husband having Alzheimer's disease, but I do know my faith in Christ was strengthened.

I kept reminding myself that Jesus had not promised to change the circumstances of my life, but He had promised me peace and joy, if I would follow Him. And I tried to remember that acceptance comes before understanding.

During those long years as we wandered in the valley, I rode an emotional roller coaster, One day I would wake up optimistic, and the next day be down in the dumps. Some days it was easier to deny the possibility of death looming in the near future. If will power and desire had been enough, we would have conquered Alzheimer's disease, but we all know that is not possible. My husband was not afraid of death, but he did not want to die.

"This road ends in the cemetery" reads a sign on a dusty country road in Oklahoma. The truth, of course, is that all life ends in the cemetery and if we don't enjoy the scenery and smell the roses along the way, we will have missed out on what is truly important. Enjoying life's scenery is not easy when we constantly live with the specter of death by our side.

One day when Herrick had fallen in the driveway while I was helping him out of the car, and I had to call for help to get him inside, he was terribly upset. He understood enough of what was happening to him to be embarrassed. After I got him settled inside in his chair, he spent two hours mumbling and saying over and over, such things as:

> I'm no good to anybody anymore.
> I don't want to be here anymore.
> I love all of you
> No one thinks I'm any good
> What use am I anyway.
> I guess no one likes me now.

At such times as this I know he was aware of what he was saying. The night following this episode, he suffered hallucinations with chills and shaking.

58

The next morning his speech was slurred and he was drowsy. This was the beginning of the seizures or TIA's which became more and more frequent. As noted in my journal for that day, he was alert in the afternoon and told me I was the best there was and asked if I liked him anymore. I told him, of course, I liked him and hugged and kissed him. He laughed out loud, for the first time in weeks, and put his arms around me and said, "This is the best ever," the phrase he always used when he was especially pleased

Skippy, his puppy, had been his constant companion for four years. As the disease progressed, I noticed Herrick would become irritated with her when she tried to sit in his lap or on the chair beside him. Obviously, he no longer found pleasure in having her around. Since it was becoming more difficult for me to find time to take care of Skippy, I made the difficult decision to find her a new home. After she was gone, he asked about her only one time. I told a "white lie" and said she was outside. He seemed satisfied with that answer and never asked about her again.

Caring for a loved one with Alzheimer's disease is not simply a grieving process; grief becomes a way of life. I learned to carry a pocket full of Kleenex because I never knew when I would start crying.

As we realize that our days together are indeed numbered, it does cause sadness. However, it is also our opportunity to consider each day a gift and determine to make it special in some little way.

A year or so before the end, Herrick would sometimes think I was his sister, or his mother. I would tell him I was Dorothy, his wife, and he would ask where his mother was. When I explained that she was in heaven with Jesus and that he would soon be going there and could see her, he would accept my explanation and be content.

It is not uncommon for those in the late stage of Alzheimer's to confuse their caregiver with a loved one from the past. I learned it was best to ignore it when he called me by another name. He could not have understood if I corrected him. I would answer to whomever he thought I was, as I sensed it was meaningful to him to think that person was with him.

Since he no longer watched TV and had already forgotten his dog, he would just sit and stare into space unless I was talking to him or feeding him.

Quite by accident, I discovered that if I gave him a basket of his socks and asked him to match and fold them for me, he would stay occupied for 30 to 45 minutes. Of course, the socks were mismatched, but that was not the purpose for the activity. I began giving him towels and wash clothes to fold. He would fold, refold and fiddle with them for long periods of time. Through these exercises, he felt useful and needed.

As he began sleeping more and more, I wondered if that was his way of escaping what he could no longer understand. I was torn between trying to keep him awake and alert and letting him sleep. But since nothing interested him anymore, what else was he to do but sleep? I felt it was kinder to let let him sleep, thereby escaping the world he could no longer understand.

Chapter 11

Enduring to the End

~~~~~~

What cannot be cured,
can be endured.
-William James

My daily routine was to tell myself that all I needed to do was get up and make it through just that one day; tomorrow would take care of itself.

There were mornings when I did not want to drag myself out of bed. After a pep talk with myself, and a prayer asking God for strength, I would get up. And once things were underway, the routine kept me going.

Often I had debates with myself about which was worse for him, letting him be terribly confused and miserable because he was lost and thought people were persecuting him, or keeping him semi-sedated with anti-anxiety drugs.

I never administered as much pain medication as his doctors had indicated I safely could, but I did not withhold medicine either. My goal always was to keep him relaxed, but not sedated.

The delusions about family members trying to hurt or kill him would come out of nowhere at the most unexpected times. I could find nothing in his early years before I knew him which might have triggered these thoughts. I knew for certain there was nothing in the 55 years I had known him which would account for his fears.

The delusions did not seem to have any factual basis whatsoever. In talking with other caregivers, I find this type of behavior is not uncommon for the Alzheimer's patient.

Low grade fevers with chills and shaking began to occur more and more often. Following the chills he would get sweats so heavy I would have to change his night clothing and the bed linens. Each time following these episodes, he would be physically wiped out, not wanting to eat or even take juice. Even if I managed to get him up and dressed the day following these episodes, he would almost always want to go right back to bed.

Whether these sweats and chills were caused by the disease, the doctors could not say

One morning, shortly after he had gone back to bed, he called to me. I went to him and he wanted to know if he was dying, which caught me off guard.

I was momentarily speechless. But I took his hand, told him we would all die some day, but it was up to God when that would be. I also said that I did not think it would be that day or even next week, but when we did die, we would go to heaven to be with Jesus and our loved ones. He listened to what I said, then asked if I would go with him when he went.

If at any time during my caring for my husband in our home, I had thought he would be getting better care in a nursing home, I would have placed him. Two years before his death I put his name on a waiting list. Each time there was a vacancy and they called me, I considered the pros and cons but always backed off. It was as if God was telling me to wait; it was not yet time.

If he had been in a nursing home, I believe he would have known he was not in his "comfort zone" and would have been more agitated and confused. I am so grateful to God that he gave me the physical and mental strength needed to care for Herrick at home.

Caring for your loved one at home is not for everyone. Sometimes it is best for everyone involved if the loved one is placed in either assisted living or a nursing home. Quality of life is what you are seeking for them, and if this cannot be accomplished by keeping them at home, then you do what is best for them. Again, everyone and each circumstance is different and each person must make this determination for himself

Early on when he was in the hospital for treatment, my husband said, "You know this is not the way it is supposed to be," meaning he did not want to be institutionalized. I felt my marriage vows "for better or for worse" should apply as long as I was able to care for him.

I remember reading somewhere that God provides a path through, not a bridge over, our troubles. He certainly provided a path through this dark valley for me. I endured what would have seemed impossible if I had seen the whole picture at the beginning of our ordeal. God knew that if taken one day at a time, it was possible.

Chapter 12

Never Losing Faith

~~~~~~

***"Love never gives up, never loses faith,
is always hopeful, and endures through
every circumstance"***
-I Corinthians 13:7

As the months passed and he began dragging his feet, barely able to walk, I walked in front of him pulling the walker. He began to forget how to pick up and move the walker. Even after installing wheels, he could not remember to push it. I realized he was close to becoming bedfast.

As long as I could I kept him with me in our bedroom. I knew it would not be long before he would have to use the hospital bed, and the only place for a hospital bed in our small house was in the den. I wanted to be with him as long as we could make it work. Not being able to share a bed after 50 plus years of marriage was painful to consider.

The time came when I could not safely move him from his chair and down the hall to our bedroom. So the hospital bed which he had been using for daytime naps, became his nighttime bed as well.

To help make the transition from sleeping together to being alone, I would lie beside him on the small hospital bed until he was asleep. We both needed this closeness. Many nights I would fall asleep only to wake up an hour or so later barely hanging on the side of the bed.

Shortly after that change, it became a challenge for me to get him safely from the bed to his lift chair, which we had purchased after his stroke. He was fast losing strength in his legs, and some times fell, even though I kept close watch on him.

He complained of pain in his head, legs or back, and would say, "Help me, please." Often the pain medication would not help him because these pains were emotional/mental for the most part. I suffered right along with him.

There will be times that, try as you might, you will be unable to make your loved one comfortable or happy. The feelings of helplessness and anguish are tough for caregivers. I discovered that sitting with him, holding his hand as we listened to quiet music, was sometimes more successful in quieting him than the medications were.

For some time I had needed cataract surgery but kept postponing it because I did not want to upset my husband by leaving him with others for a whole day. Finally when my vision affected my driving, I knew it was foolish to postpone surgery any longer.

When I returned home from the day surgery with a patch over my eye, he was quite upset and kept wanting to pull it off. He thought someone had hurt me and said he was going to kill the person who had done it. He remained agitated and restless, mumbling incomprehensive words, all afternoon, not calming down until long past bed time.

That night as I lay beside him in the hospital bed, he took hold of my hand, saying he did not want anyone hurting me. The patch on my eye had affected him so much he kept remembering it.

Any changes around our loved ones affects their mental state. It is important that everything remain as routine as possible, but be aware and prepared when the routine has to be changed.

As soon as he began spending nights in the hospital bed, I purchased baby monitors, which worked great for us. I could relax and sleep, confident I would be able to hear him if he woke up and needed me. Like a mother with a new baby, I was always alert and would hear any unusual sound and instantly be awake.

I highly recommend monitors to anyone who sleeps in a room separate from their care partner. The monitors also come in handy during the day when you have to be in a different room and need peace of mind that all is well with your loved one.

One night I was awakened around midnight by his talking. When I went into his room and asked what was wrong, he said, "I was looking for you." I had been with him when he fell asleep, and for whatever reason he woke up and missed me. I lay down beside him placing my arm across his chest, and told him I was still there with him. He thanked me and went back to sleep.

Many nights he would wake up and just need the assurance that someone was with him. Having this feeling of closeness was a security for him, and I believe it helped keep his fears at bay.

Each day when our mail was delivered, I read aloud the notes and cards from relatives and friends. He may not have understood everything I said, but he would listen and mumble, "That's nice." Since he would not be able to remember from one day to the next, I could and did read them over and over. He liked to look at the pictures on the cards and I talked to him about the friends, or relatives, who had sent them.

At night I would read to him from the Bible, then recite the 23rd Psalm or the Lord's Prayer before we went to sleep. He would lie still and listen to every word. During his restless periods in the afternoon I would sit with him and read poetry which had a calming effect on him. I would read slowly so that if possible he could understand and comprehend what I was reading. During these times I held his hand and sometimes he squeezed back, but most of the time he would lie with his eyes closed.

At times he fell asleep before I finished reading to him. At other times, if he was restless and not ready for sleep when I was through reading, I would sit by his bed and talk to him. When I got weary I would lay my head beside his on the pillow. It was not unusual for me to fall asleep like this, waking up a while later when my neck got tired.

According to my journal it was around this time that Herrick's chanting about going home and wanting his mother would get so bad that neither quiet music, nor my talking to him helped. The doctor had instructed me on how much medication to give at these times.

About a week prior his being admitted to the hospital with pneumonia, he developed a bad cough and started running a low grade fever. Like a child, he kept asking for his mother. He would not eat, and I had to coax him to get him to drink a little juice or water.

The cough did not let up and he became so miserable I called the doctor. After describing the symptoms, especially the cough, the doctor prescribed cough medicine and an antibiotic.

Just two days later in the early evening his temperature spiked to 103 and the cough persisted. I called 911 and had him taken to the emergency room where pneumonia was diagnosed and he was admitted to the hospital.

Deep down I knew this event signaled the beginning of the end, that physically he could not cope with pneumonia. His pain was so severe that my only concern was to somehow relieve his pain. After all he had already suffered, I would have gladly given anything if I could have taken his pain upon myself.

After one week of hospitalization the doctor told the family the pneumonia was not responding well to treatment, and suggested we consider Hospice if we wanted to bring him home. The alternative was a nursing home.

Having to make this decision was a sad time for us. Either my daughter or I spent every hour with him at the hospital. I stayed days and some nights. She had a job and needed to get some sleep. I grew weary but amazingly I was not so tired that I was unable to keep alert and act responsibly as his advocate.

I learned that even the best managed and best run hospitals cannot always give adequate attention to their patients. They simply do not have enough personnel. I found that medicines were not always administered on time; patients who were in pain but unable to tell the nurse were overlooked; and prompt attention for personnel hygiene needs were not always a priority. Being there day and night I was able to help with Herrick's care.

Eventually you will have to become your loved one's advocate in a medical setting. Be respectful, but firm, when you see a need not being met.

As we began the second week of hospitalization, Herrick said he wanted to go home and he wanted me to go with him. I have wondered if he might have overhead our discussions with the doctor about nursing home vs. hospice. I hope that was not the case.

Once again he told me he did the best he could. After two weeks in the hospital we came home under Hospice care. I thought I was prepared for the words "hospice" and "end of life," but discovered I was not as prepared as I had thought.

About this time the TV documentary on death and dying by Judith and Bill Moyers was aired. Watching this program helped me a great deal in finding peace with our decision to place him under Hospice home care. His speech was slurred and he had difficulty enunciating words caused either by the TIA's or pain medication.

Deciding on Hospice was not easy. However, there comes a time when a decision must be made as to whether what we are doing is prolonging life or just delaying death.. When life becomes a burden to the one who is sick, and needs mechanical intervention to stay alive, I believe it is time to stop delaying death.

Years before the diagnosis of Alzheimer's disease, Herrick and I had each executed our Living Wills. So making decisions about mechanical intervention, feeding tubes or heroic efforts was not one the family had to make. Herrick had already made that decision.

Everyone, whether they have Alzheimer's disease or not, should have Living Wills, Durable Powers of Attorney and Medical Powers of Attorney in place.

Once a person is diagnosed with Alzheimer's disease, or some other form of dementia, it is difficult to get these done. And in time, it will be necessary that someone be authorized to speak for the impaired person.

Once we were home from the hospital under Hospice care and knew we would not be taking him back to the hospital, the rest fell into place. No heroic measures would be taken to sustain life. We would not withhold food or water, nor regular medicines especially pain medication, but when these could no longer be taken orally, we would not use forced tube feeding, nor intravenous methods.

Using Hospice was one of the best decisions I made for Herrick's care. Medicines were given for comfort and for the most part we were able to keep him free of pain for the fifteen months he was under Hospice care.

It is easy to overlook the reality that none of us will live on this earth forever. We are all going to die. Earth is our temporary home. As Christians we believe heaven is our destiny. Toward the end of his life on this earth, my husband barely existed in any conscious way. Truly, he hovered between two worlds.

Watching him in this state was extremely difficult to bear. I prayed that since it had not been God's will to return him to a healthy state, He would take my husband to his heavenly home. I felt peace praying this, because I knew deep in my heart that Herrick would want it that way.

As he became totally dependent on me and others, I could occasionally see that he was aware of his condition, and how sad it made him. One day as I changed his wet clothes and bed, he mumbled softly, "I can't do this anymore." How heart wrenching that he had to undergo this indignity.

Chapter 13

Hard Things Get Harder

~~~~~~

The worst thing is never the last thing.
-Unknown

One of the worst things about Alzheimer's disease
is not having your lifetime companion remember the
good times you shared. The companionship is gone
even before they die. Their past is wiped out of their
memories.

From reading the Bible I remember that both
Jeremiah and Paul told their stories of pain and hurt.
Jeremiah told his to God and Paul told his to trusted
friends. Could I do any less? When hard things get
harder we bear up by telling our story.

Talking with friends and sharing my deepest
feelings with God through prayer was my way of
dealing with my pain. There were times I would sit and
talk with my husband about trips we had taken or times
spent with our children. I do not know if he
understood any of what I was saying, but just sitting
with him and talking helped me.

During this period of his illness the tired days
flowed into each other without any let up at all. Jesus
told us to cast our care on Him and He would care for
us. Without claiming this precious promise each day I
would not have made it through the last few painful

weeks. Those who have faith can lean on a higher power and receive strength to help get through times such as this.

Six months before Herrick's death, I noted in my journal: "Horizons have shrunk. Priorities have changed and continue to change daily as the need dictates. There is very little "me" time, but that is what is needed at the moment. I can do it. Each year for the past several years has been different and each in its own way more difficult. But none so difficult as this one."

My husband never called me by name anymore, but there were moments when I am sure he knew who I was. A few times he would murmur, "Love you" and those are precious memories.

Being able to hear those whispered declarations of love were worth the effort of caring for him 24 hours a day, seven days a week. It seemed that as each failure occurred, there would be a short period of time when he would be more alert, almost as though by will power.

The days he spent lying on his hospital bed staring out the picture window, I actually felt his spirit slipping away. Can one person's thoughts create vibrations in the atmosphere to such an extent that another close to them can pick up on these vibrations? I think so. Especially for those who are close, such as a couple who has spent a lifetime together.

Seizures began occurring frequently during the last few months and each was frightful for both of us. The changes in his brain were now evidencing themselves with physical symptoms.

Stomach upsets became so bad that eating was painful for him. Sometimes just turning him in bed would upset him. He would tell me or the CNA to go away and leave him alone. One day as I tried to comfort him I suddenly began crying. I cried so hard for about five minutes that it was hard to breathe. Nothing in particular precipitated this, but simply a buildup of emotional sadness which needed release.

These releases of emotional tension serve a purpose. They relieve stress. You should never be ashamed to cry. Be honest about your feelings.

Just because you have taken on the role of caregiver does not mean you are any less a feeling, human being. Releasing tension is a healthy thing to do.

Though my husband lay barely ten feet from me I was for all practical purposes alone. He would mumble a few words when I spoke to him, but nothing made sense. Feeling overwhelmed, I began trying to live by "One thing at a time; first things first, and nothing has to be perfect." That was how I made it through each day.

I had to work to make myself take only one step at a time and give no thought to the next. It helped to remember that tomorrow's problems can safely be left to tomorrow.

The advocacy role did not disappear under Hospice care, just changed. Once when a new medication was prescribed for painful bladder spasms, Herrick began sleeping constantly. I could not wake him to eat. When I asked, both the pharmacist and nurse said it could not possibly be caused by the medication. When I questioned the meaning of XL following the name of the medicine and found it meant time release, I knew I had been right in suspecting the medicine since he chewed all his pills and had been getting the total effect all at once.

What could the doctor and pharmacist have been thinking? Both knew he chewed his pills. Since my husband was just one of many patients I suppose this detail merely slipped by them. I learned from this experience that I had to be the one responsible for my husband's well being.

When nursing assistants would fail to show up as scheduled or the nurse needed to reschedule, I was understanding. I knew there were other patients to be seen, and emergencies occurred, but caring for my husband was my concern. I was not beyond pleading, cajoling, urging and sometimes demanding when it became necessary in order to get help for him.

I tried always to be respectful, but learned how to be firm. As long as there was communication we could work around any issue. Many times, there was never any notice that someone would not be coming as scheduled, and that left me waiting without knowing what was happening . The caregiving role is stressful enough without such scenarios. Establishing communication with your auxiliary caregivers early on is vitally important

Herrick's physical condition worsened daily and I was challenged trying to keep up with these changes. When the cough returned, possibly signally the return of pneumonia, I was torn as to whether to administer antibiotics or not. We had been told by his doctors that it was not a question of if pneumonia would return, but when.

In my heart I knew my husband would not want his life prolonged under these painful conditions, when there was no possible hope for a cure.

At this time my blood pressure went sky high for the first time in my life. Since I had never had this problem previously, both my doctor and I knew it was stress related and decided to control it without medication.

I made it a point to take five to ten minutes each hour or so to relax, take deep breathes, and meditate or pray. Along with this practice, and watching my salt intake, I was able to get the pressure back to a safe range. I also made a determined effort to put things in balance. There was no need to rush all the time trying to get everything done. If it was not related to my husband's comfort, I decided it could wait. I took time to sit on the deck listening to the quiet and letting nature nourish my soul.

The coughing continued, and Herrick seemed to go inside himself. I could hear him whispering, but could not make out much of what he was saying. Every now and then I could hear him whisper his sister or brother's name. As he was doing this, his hands were in constant motion. All his life he "talked with his hands" so this seemed to be a normal action. This talking to someone only he could see continued for several days, and for him it was real.

Chapter 14

Letting Go

~~~~~~

"Love can never lose its own"
-John Greenleaf Whittier

An entry in my journal says: "I must strive to remember God loves Herrick more than I do. God gave His son for my husband, and I just give up a few hours sleep."

Gradually food and liquid intake become less and less and Herrick's weight loss became quite noticeable. He had problems getting his mouth open, and when he did take a bite, there were problems swallowing. Pureeing and mashing his food or giving nourishment in liquid form became a necessity. Ensure and fruit juices comprised most of his diet. Since he took little nourishment at any one time, I feed him four to six times a day.

Bad news of any kind, like the death of a cousin, or diagnosis of cancer for a close friend, had the power to throw me into a deep sadness. I realize now that what I was experiencing was premature grieving for the loss I knew I would soon be experiencing.

The seizures began increasing and were more severe. After each one, I would sit and talk with him, sometimes playing soft music. As I held his hand he would gradually relax and go to sleep. I am so thankful I was able to be there for him when the seizures came because I could sense his fear, and he needed someone to reassure him and hold his hand.

Since he was unable to communicate his pain, I would watch his facial expressions and try to gauge when he was uncomfortable and needed pain medication. For someone who had been self reliant all his life, it was so sad to see him at the mercy of others to provide the most basic comforts for him. He was always easy to get along with throughout our marriage, and in these awful circumstances, he still was.

Painful bladder spasms caused me to make the decision to remove the catheter. The nurse expressed doubt that he would be able to void if it were removed, but because of his pain, I decided to take the chance since it had bothered him from the time it was placed. He was able to do without it, and was much more comfortable. I did not mind the extra work of changing Depends, or changing an occasional wet bed.

A doctor friend from out of state came to visit us a couple of times to see if there was some way he could be of help. Each time he came, he would assure me that Herrick was getting the best care possible where he was, and if only I would take care of myself, I would be able to take care of my husband until the end. These words were most reassuring.

As the coughing continued, and the fever elevated, I knew it meant another bout with pneumonia, and I made the decision that we would not administer antibiotics this time. He had been through enough already, and it was time to let him go when the pneumonia returned.

As the coughing and his fever accelerated, he began mumbling more and more. Was it possible he was trying to tell us something? We don't know, but I did try to stay close by him throughout the day. And I never left his side until he was asleep for the night.

Food intake became practically nothing. Getting any liquids down was a daily struggle. He began to drift in and out of consciousness.

Occasionally he would be alert and lucid. On one such afternoon, which I recorded in my journal as being a "good time for both of us," I sat with him and told him I loved him and asked did he know that? This time against all odds, he smiled and said, "Sure" all the while holding my hand and rubbing his thumb across the back of my hand. I am positive he was totally in the present during that hour or so. On another day shortly afterwards, I again said, "You know I love you, don't you?" Very clearly he answered, "Of course." Nothing can take these memories from me.

During those hours I believe he knew he was dying. At one time he mumbled "Will you go with me?" He was restless and his eyes searched for me when I got out of his sight. When friends came to visit he attempted to talk, but couldn't form any words, just looked at them with a questioning expression.

Shortly before he died, unusual things began to happen. One day when he was quite restless, and I cranked his bed to a sitting position, he looked out the window beside the bed and exclaimed, "There are two of them!" Startled by his uttering words I could understand, as much as what he had said, I rushed to him asking who they were. He did not answer, just closed his eyes and either went to sleep or pretended to. Just what did he see? Angels, departed loved ones, or was he only hallucinating? Who is to say?

Chapter 15

The Big Picture

~~~~~~

"In truth it is life that gives unto life—while
you, who deem yourself a giver, are but a witness"
—Kahlil Gibran

I had to keep reminding myself that my circumstances didn't matter, but God's purpose did. God knew about my circumstances and was concerned with my well being, but He was more concerned with transforming me spiritually because His perspective is eternal. Nothing touches my life that He is not aware of, and tribulations can be vehicles for God's purpose.

Being a caregiver can be a blessing, as well as a burden. Caregiving means I don't always have the answer or know what is best, and it means I have to own up to my fears and shortcomings. Being a caregiver has shown me my weaknesses and my strengths. In the areas where I was the weakest, I found growth and strength.

As I shared my feelings and the issues I was facing with others in my support group, I found hope and strength to complete the journey. Support groups do just that, support each other and provide the extra encouragement needed.

I began sleeping on a cot beside his bed so I could hold his hand or lay my head on the bed beside him during the night if he stirred. I did not get much rest during those last days, but I didn't seem to be any the worse for it. We indeed do find strength when we need it. Once when I got up to use the bathroom, he mumbled "Don't go" so I knew for a certainty he was aware of my presence.

As his breathing became shallow, even with the oxygen, which he had been on for a few weeks, and his heartbeats became irregular with low blood pressure, the Hospice nurse told me his time was very near. She asked if I was ready to let him go. My answer was that I was as ready as I would ever be. I doubt any of us are really ready to lose our dear ones.

If we spoke his name and called to him, he would open his eyes temporarily, then go right back to sleep. I knew that his death could not be far off since he had stopped eating, and it was more and more difficult to get him to take liquids.

My mind knew, and I clearly understood, that he would be better off, if he went home to his eternal rest, but my heart kept resisting. His last attempt to talk to me was to say, "I have to tell you..." but then he could not finish. Taking a chance on what he was trying to say, I told him I loved him too, and thanked him for telling me. A half smile crossed his face and even if that was not what he intended to say, I know my words pleased him.

Each night as I went to bed for my two to three hours sleep before having to get up to reposition him, my prayer would be, "Lord, give me deep, restful sleep for these next two hours, so I am rested enough to care for him." And I always found it to be so. The only difference from one day to the next was whether the aide or the nurse appeared.

Two special days occurred during his last few days on earth. Thanksgiving and our 55th wedding anniversary. Some of our children came for dinner on each occasion, and I used our good china and made the dinners as festive as possible. Even though he could not physically join us at the table, he was still present a few feet away in his bed.

Chapter 16

Death is not the End

~~~~~~

Life is eternal. Love is immortal.
Death is nothing save the limit of our sight.

The day the nurse suggested Herrick was clinging to life because he sensed I was not yet ready to say goodbye was a defining moment for me.

Painful though it was, I told him I understood how he was suffering and it was all right for him to let go. I would be joining him in the near future and I would be all right in the meantime. It was amazing, but he did relax and his breathing became easier. The nurse was probably right. She had seen many similar instances.

Keeping nightly vigils beside his bed became my habit the last few days of his life. I would talk to him and recite Scripture such as the 23rd Psalm, never knowing if he heard me since he was either in a coma, or unconscious. He might not even have been aware of my presence, but it was a comfort to me anyhow.

One night while sitting with him, I wrote his obituary.

His last night was both a nightmare and a precious memory. I talked with him, rubbed his back and for a little while lay beside him on the hospital bed hugging him. A couple of times I drifted off to sleep only to wake up when his breathing became ragged. One of our daughters and his favorite aide was with us when he drew his last breath early the next morning.

Friends shared with me later that they "knew" when he had died. Saying they had "felt" his passing and were at that very moment praying for his release from his pain.

The last few weeks of my husband's life were extremely difficult. Yet I had a majestic feeling like I was somewhere between heaven and earth. Perhaps my spirit was joining his as he drifted further toward the end of his earthly life, a perfect harmony of our spirits. Just as our two life forces had been joined as one for so many years, we both knew we were about to be parted. I was so much more aware of everything during those last days. In a way this awareness was his last gift to me.

Those who have known great love, experience great pain at parting. Such is the price we pay for that love. I know I will be united with him again some day, but in the meantime, life goes on for me.

Now I must find something worthwhile and productive to do with my life after these years of caregiving. While we cannot stop the difficulties of life, we can choose how we respond. The life we will live following caregiving is the life we choose.

Amid the grief following my husband's death, I felt

92

peace and comfort knowing I had accomplished my goal, which from the outset of our journey through Alzheimer's, was to live each day so there would be no regrets at the end. I had realized this goal.

My experience has taught me that caring for the ending of life is just as precious as caring for the beginning.

Celen Keller in *We Bereaved* said, "When one door of happiness closes another opens, but often we look so long at the closed door that we do not see the one which has opened for us." Moving beyond caregiving is something we caregivers have to learn to do.

I am confident that in time I will be able to turn loose of the past and look toward the future. Until that time, however, I will do as John Greenleaf Whittier wrote in the following:

No longer forward nor behind
I look in hope or fear;
But grateful, take the good I find
The best of now and here.

You, too, can do it—one day at a time.

Following is a poem I wrote shortly after my husband's death:

Empty Rocking Chair

Two rocking chairs sit side by side
One chair is empty, one is occupied.
They sit on the porch where they've been for years
They've seen much laughter, but also some tears.

Now one chair is empty, its occupant gone.
The other chair holds the one left alone.
The empty chair waits, it neither knows nor cares
Death claimed the one who sat there for years.

But the one left behind rocking to and fro
Knows and remembers the one she loved so.
And though she is sad, she's not really grieving,
She knows before long she, too, will be leaving.

Dorothy C. Snyder
© 2002

About The Author

The author is uniquely qualified to write about caregiving. Her husband suffered from Alzheimer's disease and she cared for him at home until his death.

Writing from personal experience, she does not hesitate to show her vulnerability in an effort to encourage and inspire those who are on the caregiving journey with a loved one who suffers from Alzheimer's disease. She pulls no punches in telling her story with the hope that it will encourage and inspire other caregivers.

Snyder is the author of numerous articles which have been published in several periodicals and magazines.